First and foremost, I would like
to thank God for allowing me
to go through the dark so that I
can come out in the light! To
my mother, Arnetta
Livingston, I love you so much!
Thank you for raising me and
teaching me to be the best man
I could be. To all my sisters,
thank you for always
encouraging me throughout
my journey. I love you all

-Glen

A Dream Catchers Publication ©

The Naked Truth

As I sit here and
reflect on my childhood,
many thoughts begin to
run through my head.
Some good and some
bad. There are some
memories that I try to

forget about, but my

weight has been a topic

that has always

presented a dark cloud

for me. Since a young

child, I've always had

issues with myself and

the way I appeared. My

peers always asked,

"How could you be so active yet so big"? But to be honest, I really had no clue why. I would just laugh it off and change the subject, hiding my true feelings. I was on the football team, double-dutch, step team, and I even ran track and field. I

remember jumping rope

on Hoe Avenue in the

Bronx and the drug

dealers would yell "Look

at big boy". How in the

world was I still so big!

I come from a particularly large family. Having five sisters and me being the only boy, whatever my sisters did, I followed and succeeded. My mother and sisters taught me to always be great. But I honestly loved food and still do!

While my mother cooked

dinner some nights, I

would sit in the kitchen

with her, throwing

tantrums. I would tell her

to hurry up before I die of

starvation. She would

always reply with "son,

it's coming". I was a complete spoiled brat. My sisters would spoil me by taking me to the store and telling me to get whatever I wanted. I would pile on all the cakes and cookies I could find. My face would literally light up as I ate my snacks. My grandmother always said "a full boy is still a boy".

As a child, I didn't fully understand why my family loved me so much. I was fat and miserable. It was as though they couldn't even notice that I was overweight. In fact, my family actually loved my size. My oldest sister would always say "That's my big Glen". My youngest sister loved that I was her protector as we walked to school. My

sister, Nasha was the

only one who really knew

my naked truth about

how I really felt, although

I had never expressed

my issues to her.

On the outside, I

appeared fine to

everyone else. But on the inside, I was dying. I was miserable and was constantly bullied because of my weight. Sometimes, I would have to even wear my step father's clothes to school because I couldn't fit my own and people knew it!

Being 235 pounds in the

sixth grade was not an

easy issue to deal with.

Even at this tender age, I

had a reputation to

uphold so I would fight

anyone who negatively

spoke about me just to

protect my own feelings about myself. Even if a person just looked at me the wrong way, I would swing before those words could even leave their mouths. You know.. fat boy! I didn't feel good nor look good to anyone who seen me outside. Instead, people would use me because of my weight. If any of my friends had a problem, I was their go-to fighter.

One day, I found myself so fed up over the bullying and I bought a knife to school. I swear I didn't want to use it but I had to end the negative words thrown at me from these three boys. They constantly attacked me about my weight. I had seen them right after the bell signaled that school was over and I

completely blacked out.

All I can remember is

walking home crying

because I had stooped so

low to stop people from

bullying me.

Although my weight

never stopped me from

doing anything, as I grew older, I stopped myself. But silly me, I thought. My weight definitely stopped me one day at an amusement park. This was the biggest wake up call of my life! I was on a date and I couldn't even fit on the ride. What broke

me down completely was

that I had to walk back

through the long line of

people who were waiting

to actually get on the ride.

So here I was, standing

there while my date was

on the ride, trying to hide

my true feelings about

what had just happened.

    If you thought the

date was bad, you

haven't heard the worst

yet! I will never forget my

first day of music class in

high school, I got stuck in

the chair! My weight had

become out of control as I hit 300 pounds. My mother went school shopping for me and could no longer figure out my size. So I squeezed myself into the tightest pair of jeans on the first day of school. It was the first day, c'mon I had to look fly too! At the end of the period, I attempted to get up and the entire desk followed my lead. I heard the laughter of my classmates and the embarrassment rose. After that, there was days where I wouldn't even eat school lunch because I knew people would be staring at me like an animal at the zoo.

Not long after my mom had moved to North Carolina, I got a phone call that shook me to my core. My mother was always optimistic and so positive towards life. But this day was different. She told me that the doctor had just informed her that she had stage four cancer. My heart skipped multiple beats as

I just stood their silent.

After a minute of silence

she said, "but I know God

got me son". This was

when I moved to North

Carolina. I just had to be

near my mother. I would

rush home to her every

night, praying for and with

her. I would continue to encourage her that God would heal her. But the cancer only began to worsen. A week after our last conversation, my mother passed away. After that, I fell into a really bad depression.

And I would separate

myself from everybody.

This was when food

really became my rock.

All I did was eat! I was

now 383 pounds and my

only best friend was

Chinese food. My friend

Amanda would bring me

shrimp fried rice with chicken wings, a side of crab sticks and sugar doughnuts every day! Oh, and let's not forget the 3-4 packs of gummy worms a day on top of everything. My shirts were a 6x and even that was tight for me. I always wondered why the stores didn't sell bigger sizes for people like me. I literally stuffed myself with food. I watched my stomach stretch before my eyes.

One night, I remember asking God to

take my life. Without my mother, I felt as though I really had no purpose for living. Losing her made me feel as though I had jumped off the roof of a building and I was waiting to hit the pavement. I could literally feel myself in the air falling, but the pavement was still so far away. This was when I knew something had to change.

The next day I woke up and declared to myself that enough was enough.

It was time to take my life back! I went to the doctor and broke down crying about everything, and she cried with me. I just remembered her telling me that this was no way to live. She asked me what I wanted and I just kept screaming "HELP"!

She told me that I was

suffering from anxiety

and prescribed me

Wellbutrin. Wellbutrin is a

type of antidepressant

that also acts as a

stimulant. But the side

effects were terrible!

Nausea, vomiting, dry mouth, headaches, and the list goes on! This also was a big push for me to lose weight. So over the next few days, I wrote down a list of things I wanted for my life. At the top of the list was to

move back to New York,
and next was to lose
weight. I gave myself six
months to move and I
started to decrease my
food intake, limiting my
portion size. With only
three months into my new
goals, I had lost 40

pounds and I no longer needed the medication. My doctor was so elated with the vast progress I was making. I drank nothing but water and walked in the park every day, tracking my miles.

Before I knew it, the

weight started to fall off!

Growing up with a

religious mother, I always

knew who God was for

myself at a youthful age.

But as my weight spun

out of control, I started to

depend less on him and

my faith began to diminish. Attending church again with my best friend, Amanda helped me to regain my strength. Each week that I attended, I grew stronger and stronger. I started to sing again and enjoy the services with a smile on my face.

Now that I was losing weight, I was finally able to do workouts at home. I started by doing 20 pushups, 20 crunches, and 20 squats a day. It wasn't much, but it was all I was capable of doing

at the time. Although I

was finally happy again in

North Carolina, I was just

preparing myself for my

new life back home in

New York. That's where

my heart lied and that's

the place where I knew I

could flourish; not just for me but my entire family. So I finally left and moved back home. My weight loss journey continued as I lost 72 pounds after being back for just two months! With the more weight I dropped, the more I increased my workouts. I was now able to do 50 pushups, 50 squats, and 50 crunches three times a week.

So let's get straight into things on how I made this happen. Losing weight can be very easy and also very challenging. Some people start then they quit and this cycle can honestly continue for years. I've realized three major key points when trying to lose weight. First, your mind has to be in the right place. You have to understand that hard work leads to accomplishing your goals. Secondly, you have to understand that the beginning will be the hardest phase to overcome. You may want to throw in the towel, but hang in there. A better and healthier you is on the way. And lastly, this is NOT a diet. It causes a huge restriction on what you can and cannot have, but with this lifestyle, you can enjoy any foods you want with moderation.

This is now your own way

of living. How many times

have you looked in the

mirror and despised your

reflection? The mind is

the key to your success.

To me, I always felt like

my mind never matched

my appearance. I would say things like "this is not my real body". My whole demeanor was completely different from the defeated reflection I seen in the mirror.

I've always followed my heart, but always

seemed to fail at "dieting". I never liked using the word "diet". It was so unrealistic.

There's always a start date and end date for every potential dieter. What happens when the diet ends? Do you go back to eating fried

chicken and macaroni

and cheese three times a

week? If your answer is

yes, you will gain all your

weight back and maybe

even extra pounds. I

never dieted, I just looked

at my weight loss journey

as a lifestyle; something I'll do for the rest of my life.

I would eat when I was happy, sad, and oh, just eat because I was already overweight. My mind was weak and had become so accustomed

to living the way I've lived
for many years. Change
didn't sit right with me.
But you have to speak
things into existence and
strengthen your mind.
Encourage yourself daily
and say you can do this!

Sure, the first day or two will feel so easy. But after about a week, your body will begin to notice a change in the foods you are consuming. It is no longer receiving extra calories and you'll often find yourself saying that

you're hungry. Your body
is confused at this point,
but stand firm! It's easier
to give up than it is for
you to keep trying.
Always remember that
you will win and regain
control of your life again.

After all these years, I've come to realize that losing weight can be very doable. I thought to myself that if I stayed on this track and routine, I could do this for the rest of my life with just working out.

As the weight continued to disappear, I became eager to learn more about nutrition. So eager, that I enrolled in a nutrition course at a local college. Here is where I learned why I was dropping the weight so fast. Fruits and vegetables play a leading role in weight loss. Although fruits are carbs, they are the good carbs. Our bodies use fruits as energy, which burns right off, causing no weight gain. The same rule applies for vegetables.

It's as if our bodies thirst

for these multicolored

foods, and as soon as it

enters the body, they are

used up to provide long

lasting energy.

At this point in my life,

I went from weighing 383

pounds, to 280 pounds in less than a year without surgery! My clothes were literally hanging off of me! Instead of buying a complete new wardrobe, my father suggested that I buy multiple pair of sweatpants with drawstrings until I

reached my weight loss

goal. This is when my

confidence grew and my

social skills were better

than ever. Multiple times

a day, people would

question how did I lose

so much weight in such a short time.

During my many nights of research, I stumbled across calorie counting. Calorie counting is when you add up all the calories you intake with every single thing you eat in a day. I fell in love with this method as I found it to be very beneficial. I set myself on a limit of 1800 calories a day and the weight still continued to disappear. Upon my studies, I've discovered nutrient density. This means that you ideally want to consume foods with the best nutrition that contain the least amount of calories. Trust me, calorie counting can be extremely difficult and tedious only because you're literally counting

every single calorie you

eat! But after a few

weeks of doing it, you

become a natural at it.

My family played a

significant role in

supporting me during my

weight loss journey. But

some days they would say "Okay Glen, that's enough"!

As I began to increase my workout regime, I dropped even more weight, weighing in at a total of 160 pounds! Now I do 200 pushups,

200 crunches, and 300-

500 squats three times a

week.

    With all these years

behind me, I can truly say

that I'm happy with

myself and who I've

grown to be. At the age of

32, I've finally found love

within myself. For most of
my life, I thought love
was about someone else
loving you and being
happy in a relationship.
As a child, that was
always my main goal.
Money was never top
priority for me, but being

in love was first on the

list. For a long time, I

searched to find

happiness within people

around me. I depended

on them to make me

happy. Although I thought

I found love numerous

times, it never lasted

long. It wasn't until I began to spend time alone and really focus on the things that make me happy. Losing weight set the tone for everything that was to come. It wasn't until the weight began to shed that I realized there was more

to life than being

overweight and

miserable.

One day while

working out, I dazed off

and started to think about

how happy I now was. In

my one-bedroom

apartment, just me and my dog, Toby. I just kept thinking to myself "If nothing else exciting happens in my life, I'm more than content with who I am and where I am going". When I wake up every morning, I say a prayer and thank God

because he loved me

when I didn't love myself.

I'm valuable in his eyes

and he's now showing

me just how much of a

prize I am to him. So long

are the days of me

looking for love in

someone else. How could
I ever love others when I
hated myself? Self-love is
the best feeling in the
world. I believe you must
go through tough times in
order to break-through
and really become the
person God intended for

you to be. Self-love will

lead a person to help and

inspire others.

Sometimes we put up

with things and people

due to our own

insecurities and lack of

confidence. When you

have self-love, you begin

to give up on people and things that are no longer beneficial to you, in order to walk into your destiny!

To live a healthy lifestyle is more than your physical appearance. It means your social, emotional, and spiritual identities are now under construction in hopes of becoming the best you that you can be. When I first started my journey, I had no idea that two years later, I would be sharing my story with the world. Thinking back on it all, I was just honestly trying to lose weight. But now I see, I'm destined to help people conquer their dreams by living healthy lives too. I plan to inspire and I intend to do this for the rest of my life. My mother always told me

"You are somebody", and

she was right! So declare

that today is the day you

want to take the first

steps of your new life. Put

your best foot forward

and start living a healthier

lifestyle by getting fit just

like I did. I put my life in

this book and it's the

Naked Truth!

About The Author!

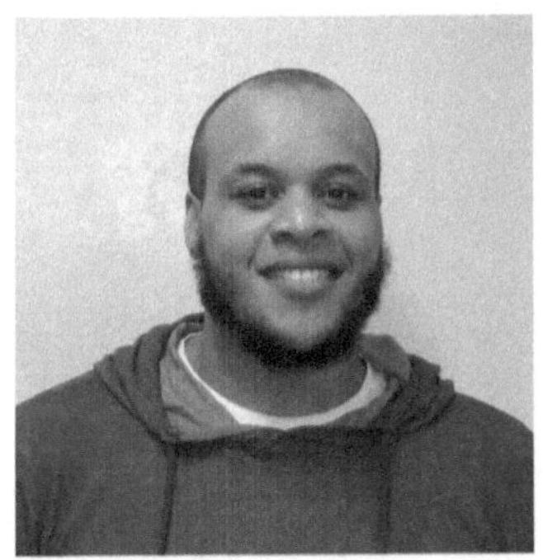

Glen Livingston was born and raised in the Bronx, N.Y. He works in the Mental Health field and is an active member at Powerhouse Cathedral United Baptist Church. Glen aspires to become a staple in the weight loss community and venture into music. He takes pride in his loving family and inspires to help others.

www.ingramcontent.com/pod-product-compliance
Lightning Source LLC
Chambersburg PA
CBHW031324250726
48656CB00005B/1958